Your Diet Success Plan

Lower Your Weight and

Elevate Your Health and Happiness

by

Changing How You View Dieting!

2nd Edition
Produced by
Caryl Hallberg
Dogwatch Navigation LLC
dogwatchnavigation.com

In Partnership with
ASC and Dapple Productions
©2019

Table of Contents

Before we start:

This is probably not the first diet book you've purchased. You may have an expectation that you are going to read a lot of marketing and sales pitch, wasting your time until the end where I will finally offer you a miracle for just a few dollars a month. You may hope that out of all of that you will still find some crumb of learning or insight.

I promise you that is not going to happen. I have no product to sell. I offer you my services to help assure you that you will meet your goals and make wiser decisions, but I have nothing to sell in this book other than those services.

The goal is to provide you with a different approach to thinking about your diet and habits. To provide you with some information based on data and fact, instead of hype.

You may be interested to know that as I wrote this book, I was on my own personal journey of a healthy lifestyle and diet. I already eat pretty well, though I have my potato chip moments. As I've aged, I find that my weight has increased but more than that how my body holds and uses the weight has changed.

My goal in researching for this book and my healthy diet coaching program is to share with you what I am learning along the way. Not everyone is a research and system builder the way I am, not everyone likes to build plans the way I do. Why not benefit from the work I've done?

My goal for health is to lose a bit of weight and regain some of the lost muscle mass that aging has snuck up on me. I want to be fit enough to truly live and enjoy the life I have built and continue building for myself. That is what I want for you as well, the physical and emotional capacity to live the life of your dreams.

If you appreciate the discussion, if you want some help with setting and achieving your desired results, great! Contact me and we will get you started on my health track program for eating wisely. Otherwise, take what you can from the following and if you have a moment let me know if it helped you think about your body, your weight, and your health differently.

Chapter 1: The Problem with Diets of the Past

It's a sad fact that most people who read this book are not on their first diet. In fact, probably most aren't on their second, third or even fourth diet. Like many of us, you're probably used to the merry-go-round of dieting, and each year, your weight creeps up higher and higher and you're breaking the wrong sort of records.

It's not your fault, unless you find out how to fix this problem and ignore the advice, choosing instead to get back on the same harmful, discouraging path you were on before.

What's wrong with the diets you've been on? A lot!

They Concentrated Heavily on Numbers

Most diets require you to do lots of math to properly understand and master them. From the calorie counting to the number of pounds it's okay to lose in a week to the inches you gained in muscle and lost in fat, and on and on – numbers swirling in your head can get overwhelming.

Some diets go even further than simple calories and have you performing math equations on every single meal you eat. Did you get the right number of carbs? Is the ratio of carbs to protein correct?

What happens when you're having to be a mathematician for each meal is that you get annoyed. You don't feel like counting and dividing and comparing and crunching numbers – so you just fly by the seat of your pants, do it all wrong, and wonder why you failed. Or maybe, like me, you get exhausted spending 10 minutes on math when you only have a 30-minute lunch break.

Your diet should be focused on your well-being and how you're feeling, not on whether you got your math facts right.

They Focused on Extremes

Diets in your past probably went from one end of the spectrum to the other. Elimination diets where they have an all or nothing mentality aren't feasible, and they aren't enjoyable.

You need to learn how to eat for life, not for 30 days or six months. In some diets, you eliminate whole food groups, sometimes surviving solely on fattening meats and foregoing healthy fruits and vegetables.

Now, does that sound like a smart thing to do to your body?

They're setting you up for failure because they're not doable for the long-term. If you look at a diet and start tallying up how many days you'll "have to do it" to lose a certain number of pounds, then it's not a good diet to be on.

You Develop a Diet Mindset

A diet mindset is crippling. If you become someone who is always thinking about dieting, talking about dieting, and planning your life around dieting, then you are not leading a pleasant life. My goal at DogWatch Navigation is that you always lead the life you want, one that brings you true meaning and joy.

Life should be about enjoying the time you spend with friends and family, about relishing the time you get to indulge in your favorite hobbies, about pursuing success and satisfaction in your career. It should be about working toward and fulfilling your dreams!

It shouldn't be an obsession with your body's faults or how you can take drastic measures to change the way you look. It should be about pursuing things that make you feel better, building habits that deliver total wellness, including mental happiness. A diet mindset isn't what that's about!

People with a diet mindset tend to do some of the following things:

They constantly announce their diet progress to their friends and family – what they're planning to do, what they're doing, what they did and where they failed.

They don't realize it, but they often become critical of friends and family who aren't following the same regimen that they are –

always verbally nitpicking other people's actions to force them to change.

They continually beat themselves up whenever they have slipups – always focusing on what they did wrong.

Instead of propping yourself up for yet another failure, and even more pounds packed onto your frame – make a commitment right now to change the way you diet!

Chapter 2: A Better Way to Succeed with Dieting

What you want, more than anything, is to just finally succeed. You're tired of failing and regaining even more weight than you had on you before you started.

In the past, you've motivated yourself for the start of your diet and you're ready to fight back against obesity. You start off great and probably thrive, watching the pounds fall off for days, weeks – maybe even months if you're one of the lucky few.

But it doesn't last. There comes a day when you're done. It starts with a few slip ups along the way. That turns into you beating yourself up for being a failure, and then one day you start to believe it, you start to think of yourself as a failure. You accept defeat and quit until next time.

This time I hope you are motivated to succeed just as you have been motivated in the past, but this time your goals are going to be different, resulting in the achievement of those goals, a sense of success, and the knowledge that you are the healthiest you can be.

Forget About a Time Span

Are you looking to lose weight for a month – right before your 20th high school reunion and then gain it back and more? Or is good health and appropriate weight something you want for a lifetime? We both know the answer to this question, so why are you considering diets that aren't doable forever?

Lifelong habits are what you're after. So, I want you to forget about how long you'll be dieting or how long it will take you to lose the weight you want to shed. I want you to just start today being a healthier person, period.

When you take the time pressure off yourself, it opens you up to a whole new world of success. It won't feel comfortable, though. After all, every diet has promises of "2 pounds per week" or "She lost 15 pounds" with the small print of *results not typical, that you like to ignore.

And what about those goals you have on your calendar? The ones like:

Lose the last 15 pounds of baby weight by May 15th

Lose 30 pounds before swimsuit season

Lose 50 pounds before my high school reunion

Lose 100 pounds before I walk down the aisle

What about those? You've put a ton of pressure on yourself with those goals. It's okay to have them, but without an end date in mind. And it's great if you do reach those goals by the date you desired but it shouldn't be part of the goal because…

What if you don't?

If you don't, there's a tsunami of disappointment and failure labeling coming your way. If you don't, there may be an extreme diet fad in your near future, as the deadline looms. This is not a healthy option.

You end up doing more harm than good. What really matters is that you become healthier, right? Once you analyze your body physically for its health needs (and yes, that may include weight loss), then you must adopt a total mind and body wellness approach.

Use a Total Mind and Body Approach

Dieting isn't just about your body's size. It's about fueling your body for all its needs and it's about working on your mindset so that you are all about self-care and not about wondering what others will think about you.

You need to approach dieting this time from head to toe, inside and out – on a physical and emotional level. This is going to be difficult for you to initially get used to, but once you do, you'll feel more powerful, and freer, than ever before.

You need to look at dietary changes that don't just help you get trim, but that help clear up your skin, help your heart function better, help you have more energy, help you get pregnant (if that's a goal), etc.

And you also need a diet that's not a diet in the traditional sense of the word. You want a way of eating. A way of feeding your body that makes it perform better for you. Something mindless that you can do without trying so hard.

Change the Word "Diet" to "Lifestyle"

The word diet can be a dirty word to some. It reminds them of being chained to a way of life that's limiting – something they dread. How about lifestyle from now on?

Instead of saying, "I can't eat that marbled steak; I'm on a diet and it has too many calories and too much fat," simply say, "Oh, I like eating in a way that is healthier for me, so I think I'll have chicken instead, but thanks!"

Instead of, "I must burn 500 calories so I can have a HoHo today," say, "I'm going to take care of my body by giving it time to move today and increase its performance."

Chapter 3: Analyze Your Current Diet Mindset

The first thing we must do, before you ever put a single bite of "diet food" into your mouth, and before you get up off the couch and get moving – is to set your mind on the correct path to success.

We must take an honest account of where you are mentally. It's kind of like how a doctor will look at stats going back three months to judge your blood sugar levels.

You don't want to be all revved up and excited to lose weight today and trick yourself into a false sense of security that "you've got this." We should get real! Let's see where you've stood over the years.

Are You Going into This Expecting to Fail?

If you have failed before, you'll probably fail again, right? Not necessarily, but with an attitude like that, your chances increase. You should go into this new lifestyle plan with expectations that you'll succeed.

I am not talking about wishful thinking, that's a very different concept.

This is about visualization, where you "see" yourself trimmer, healthier, and more energetic than ever before based on what you plan to do.

If you get on a diet plan that's too restrictive, you can look at the odds and assume right away that you're not going to stay on the plan 100% of the time. No one would. On super restrictive diets, when you have a slip-up, you label it a personal failure, and once you've done that labeling it doesn't matter if it's a small breach in the plan, you've "failed."

This failure label gives you permission to go off the deep end. Instead of just eating a snack sized Snicker bar, you're suddenly on a death-by-chocolate bender.

There's a big difference between a 45-calorie snack and a 1,400-calorie dessert – and the effect it has on your body, but you won't care because you're being so rigid with yourself that even a small error in judgement means total failure. You need to get off the seesaw of reward and punishment. Get rid of your attitude that doesn't allow you to eat differently from time to time and stop labeling things as "slip-ups" or "mistakes" as you plan your new diet lifestyle.

Another problem when you never expect success is that inevitably, you don't work as hard at the task as you would if you expected to succeed. You might not even be able to recognize that your attitude is sabotaging your effort.

If you knew right now that if you pushed yourself to work up your cardio this week and stuck to a reasonable diet plan that you'd lose every pound of weight that you wanted 100% guaranteed, you'd do it.

But instead, you might be plotting your diet in a way that just has you avoiding failure for as long as you can. You might do cardio, but not nearly as hardcore as you would if you knew you'd succeed. You might eat okay, but not do it perfectly because failure is bound to happen anyway.

Time to change that attitude of failure to one of assured success!

Have You Announced It to the World?

Traditionally, diet experts have advised people to set a goal and announce it to the world. They claimed that it made you accountable for your efforts. This should be a good thing, but it isn't. There are several reasons why it's a better idea to quietly make this decision to lose weight on your own, and to keep it to yourself, and, if you have one, your coach.

Announcing your weight loss goals does put some pressure on yourself, instead of having one person beating you up (yourself), you open the door to having everyone and their grandmother comment about what you're eating, and everything they believe you're doing wrong. Studies also show that the simple task of announcing your goals satisfies you so much emotionally that it makes your tasks harder on the real things that matter, the actual nutrition and exercise portion of your diet plan.

It's as if announcing it was all you needed to do. But don't forget the guilt you feel, and the shame, when, after announcing it to all your friends, family, co-workers and Facebook friends, you must then show them what a failure you've become when you don't achieve your wild 50 pounds in 5 weeks weight loss goals.

I know you want support, that's your reason for announcing your goals to the world. You're hoping people will cheer you on and help you get past obstacles you encounter with your eating.

And yes, part of you might even appreciate the nagging that occurs when you go to your Mom's house and try loading up on some fattening dessert, only to hear "tsk tsk" from a well-meaning loved one.

But remember that this journey you're on toward better health isn't about your friends and family – it's about you. You're the only one who needs to know this and putting pressure on your acquaintances to babysit you isn't fair to them, either. If you want real help in achieving your goals enlist a professional coach.

A good coach partners with you on achieving your goals. They act as your extra inner voice of good sense, and help you stay focused on the results and success ahead of you.

When is it okay to let people know that you're eating healthier or dieting? When they're a source of the problem. If your grandmother bakes you seven pies a week, it's a problem. She needs to be told not to do that.

If your co-workers try pushing you into attending an endless stream of office celebrations with sweets, then you might say something in passing such as, "No thanks, I'm cutting down on my sugar intake." You don't need to make a declaration of your diet plans, how much weight you plan to lose, and keep a running tally on Facebook for everyone to see of every meal you ate, each time you hit the gym, and how many calories you consumed in a 24-hour period.

There's a lot of pressure to publicize your dieting, too. There are apps that will auto-Tweet your weight each week. There's another app that tells everyone on social media when you skipped a workout at the gym.

You might as well walk around with a sign around your neck that tells everyone you meet that you need their approval to be happy because you're inviting scorn, not just applause. It is time to live to please yourself. It is time to offer yourself approval and applause.

Do You Feel Guilt Associated with Diet Slip-Ups?
This is very common. In fact, if you're dieting and "slip up" in front of people without

acknowledging your guilty feelings, people wouldn't even understand why!

Stop using words and phrases like "cheated" or "fell off the wagon." Your self-talk is the first thing you should get under control so that you can stop feeling so negative about the choices you make.

Right now, you should look at the long road ahead from this day to the rest of your life and realize that not every day has to be so regimented and restricted. Once you have the freedom to understand this concept, it makes it easier for you to have things that are outside your official diet plan without raking yourself over the coals for it.

That said, this doesn't mean your diet is now open so that you exist on nothing but donuts and brownies. But when you truly allow yourself to not feel food guilt anymore, you'll see how easy it is to indulge from time to time without turning it into an official, and unhealthy binge.

Chapter 4: Evaluate Your Existing Nutritional Intake

Before you begin making nutritional changes, you should see where you currently stand. Your goal is to identify both the habits you need to change and the habits you can feel good about keeping.

The Right and Wrong Way to Keep a Food Journal
Keeping a food journal requires two things: consistency and honesty. Without both of those, a food journal isn't going to help you replace bad habits with good ones!

You can keep a food journal on your PC, using a mobile app on your phone, or even using a traditional pen and paper approach. Some people even make video blog food journals and stick them on YouTube, though I don't recommend this for reasons explained in the last chapter.

Your goal in journaling is to record everything you eat and drink so that you can understand why you stall with weight loss and other health concerns, or why you might reach a plateau or start gaining again. It's also supposed to keep you somewhat accountable in helping you stay on track with your dietary plans.

Some people like to record everything as they eat every meal. You can record ingredients, portion sizes, caloric intake right down to the percentage of vitamins and other nutrients that the foods you eat offer.

But this might be too time consuming and daunting for many people. If your life is busy, it's okay to take a moment at the end of each day and record what you ate, as long as you don't forget about the time you went into the snack room and grabbed a croissant, or dipped into someone's candy jar on their desk.

You don't have to always keep a food diary, either. Some people like to do it forever, while others prefer to do it periodically just to help them see where their behavior is going wrong in a nutritional sense.

If you eat differently just because you're journaling, this can be a good or a bad thing. It's good if it helps you eat healthier and stick to your plan, but it's bad if the plan is so restrictive that you can't do it without monitoring yourself 24/7 like the food police.

You not only want to track your food, but the other elements that affect your nutrition. That includes where you ate -was it at the table or sitting on the couch mindlessly watching TV? It also includes how you were feeling whenever you ate.

Were you stressed and anxious (could that be why you just polished off a family sized bag of potato chips?) or were you content and eating mindlessly because you were in a comfortable mood and just wanted to feel relaxed and happy? Food diaries help pinpoint triggers for you.

Some people find that it helps to write down their food goals for the day at the beginning of each food journal entry. For example, you can jot down how many servings of grains or fruit you want to try to get into your diet.

You can even cross them off as you consume them, so that you're looking at what you do eat, rather than what you can't have. A food journal can help you figure out which foods you need help getting more of or getting less of.

A food journal won't do any good unless you go back later and read it. Look at your weight loss and other health factors for the week and then look back to see where the foods you ate helped or hurt the efforts.

Doing a food journal when you first start thinking about eating better and living a healthier lifestyle is generally a good idea. It helps paint a clear picture for you of what you are eating and how you are eating right now. The style, level of detail, amount of time spent, and medium of recording the information is entirely up to you and should fit your personality, not what one method or person says is the "right" way. If you keep one continually or periodically is entirely based on what will work for you.

This is about building your understanding and success.

Are You a Grazer or a Fueler?

Some people snack all day long; from the time they wake up and pour their first cup of coffee to the moment they slip into bed with a little before-slumber snack. This is known as a grazer. Grazers don't usually sit down to three square meals a day, breakfast, lunch, and dinner. Instead, they keep their bodies going all day long by snacking. The key is in knowing why you're snacking.

Strategically, this can be a helpful dietary plan – like those who eat 6 small meals a day rather than three large ones. But if you're snacking because you're stress eating or snacking on the wrong kinds of food all day, like propping your body up with a non-stop sugar rush, then it becomes a problem.

Fuelers are different types of eaters. They fuel up with a hearty breakfast, work all morning, and stop for more nutritional fuel at lunch, doing the same at dinnertime until the day is done.

They choose not to snack in between meals. Some people prefer this because they like how it feels to eat and fill up rather than never get that specific "full" feeling that grazing lacks.

Either way, you can lose weight and feel great. The key is in choosing healthy foods that keep hunger pangs at bay, but which don't stuff you like a Thanksgiving turkey each meal.

It might be easier for you to transition from foods that aren't as nutritionally sound to foods that offer a multitude of health benefits if you keep eating on the same schedule that you always have, at least for the time being.

You might want to switch schedules after a while if you decide to, once you're familiar with the new foods and feeling confident that you enjoy the meal plans with which you're working. You may find that your system works best on five or six meals a day, or three meals with small snacks in-between. The point here is to understand your natural tendencies, discover the best rhythms for your body. Once you know what works best for you, you will be able to establish reasonable portion control, and assure that you are eating the right combinations together to provide high efficiency for your healthy lifestyle.

What Are Your Portions Like?

Portions in America have gotten out of control when it comes to most restaurant meals. The same is true in our own homes. We put way more on our plate than we really need to fuel our bodies.

Portion recommendations differ according to your age, your weight, your gender, and whether you're pregnant or breastfeeding. Still, you need to know a starting point to see where you currently are with portions.

It might help to go ahead and fix your plate and then measure the foods so that you can see what you've been doing. Don't measure before putting them on your plate because that doesn't tell you what you've been used to doing.

You might think you've only been eating a half a cup of mashed potatoes but are shocked when you measure and realize it has been 2 ½ cups this whole time.

Do you fill your entire plate? Is it a large dinner plate? Plate sizes have grown with portion sizes in America, to help fool us into thinking we're eating a normal amount.

What about how you fill your plate? Have you noticed that the biggest portions on your plate are the meats or fats, with the grains or vegetables being the tiniest portions?

It's important to see how your plate stacks up now against the future health and wellness plate you plan to prepare as you start your healthy lifestyle on whatever diet plan you choose to follow.

Portions Tip:

As you choose your personal healthy diet your portions may differ based on the needs of your body. As a rule, to keeps things simple, using your hand for portion control can be very useful. Your fist = fruit, vegetables, pasta or rice serving Your middle finger and pointer finger together = cheese

The first joint on your middle finger = butter, mayonnaise, oil
Your thumb = peanut butter, or non-cheese dairy
The flat palm of your hand (no fingers) = meat
The cup of your palm = nuts, dried fruit

Chapter 5: What Kind of Movement Is Your Body Getting?

Some people think they're more active than they really are. Along with diet, your body needs to move to maximize the benefits of your eating plan, and help you get as healthy as possible. Let's look at three different types of lifestyles so that you can see where you currently are right now. You might be on a higher level of activity than you realize and therefore need more calories to sustain your body's energy throughout the day.

This is about finding out where you are now and deciding where you want to be for your best life in the future. This is not about right or wrong or judgement, just truth.

Extreme Sedentary Lifestyles

It takes a lot to be sedentary. Most people aren't sedentary at all, they're somewhat active, going to their jobs, grocery shopping, attending their kids' sporting events or participating in family activities.

Sedentary people sit, that's all they do. They might get up to go to the restroom, their bed, or the kitchen, but other than that, they're couch potatoes the rest of the time.

Now being home doesn't necessarily mean you're sedentary, even if you happen to sit quite a bit. If you're active around the house during the day off and on, then you get bumped up to the moderate movement category.

Try to keep a little log of the hours you spend sitting down, even if it's at a desk working in an office or from home, compared to the times when you're up moving around.

You can track a week or so, but make sure it's an average week for you, not one when you happen to have a lot going on that requires more movement than usual.

Write down what it is you like to do during your sedentary moments, too. Is it sitting and staring out the window? Reading a good book? Playing video games? Watching a good TV show or movie?

Your goal later will be to incorporate some of your favorite activities into more physical movement. For example, there are video game consoles that require movement so you're not being sedentary at all.

Moderate Movement

The moderate movement level has a different meaning. It's all about light activity, more than sedentary, but not quite hardcore exerciser. The moderate mover doesn't always work to include exercise into their daily routine, but they happen to get physical activity throughout their day.

Or, it's possible that they lead sedentary lifestyles but do work in a small amount of exercise in their day, such as a 30-minute walk around the neighborhood after dinner. Moderate movement has to do less with scheduled exercise and more with general movement throughout the day.

People who fall under this category could be students in college who walk from class to class and across campus, people who work in an office setting who are constantly getting up and down out of their chairs, or workers who have jobs where they're continually moving, like doctors or blue-collar laborers.

When you start tracking your movement, look to see if you have 120-180 minutes of movement each week. If so, even if you're not working up a complete sweat during this time, then you fall under the moderate movement category.

Exercise Elite

The exercise elite are those who are extremely active. These people don't just get more movement throughout their day due to basic decisions like walking to deliver a message instead of emailing. They move throughout the day, and work in an abundance of exercise that gets their hearts beating before each day is done.

The elite exercisers are those who are considered athletes. Do you regularly play a sport or participate in athletic events like marathons that you train for continually? If so, you're an active person, not moderately active or sedentary.

To be clear, to be heart healthy you need to move during the day and add the exercise. A marathon runner might suffer from "sitting disease" because she doesn't really move except when she is training. Heart healthy has to do less with scheduled exercise, and more with general movement throughout the day that includes a portion of the day that gets your heart pumping. Some careers require you to be highly physically active. This would include a soldier, some agriculture laborers, or other industry workers. If you get anywhere from six to 10 hours a week or more, you are considered extremely active. Make a record, like you do of your nutritional intake, of how much movement you get. Not necessarily formal exercise, because all movement is good for you, but times when you're up off the couch, putting your legs and arms in motion.

Tally up the hours to see if you qualify for moderate or extreme exercise levels and then you can choose a meal plan that helps you fuel your body. The last thing you want is to cut calories to such a deficit that you weaken your energy stores and become less active and less able to lose weight effectively.

Chapter 6: What Other Health Needs Should Your Diet Assist?

Look, only you and your medical doctor know or understand your health needs and challenges. This chapter is not meant to be medical advice or to recommend specific treatment for any condition with which you may be dealing. The thing is, though, that your lifestyle, particularly exercise and diet, do impact your health! You need to know what special or unique challenges you may face, and with the help of your primary medical care professional, you need to design your diet and exercise plan to meet those challenges.

If you haven't had a physical exam in a while, this is the perfect time to schedule one!

We know that physical activity is important for everyone. In the UK, a government sponsored report indicates that physical inactivity is the fourth leading risk factor for mortality (accounting for 6% of deaths). This follows high blood pressure (13%), tobacco use (9%) and high blood glucose (6%). Being overweight or obese is responsible for 5% of global mortality.[1]

---

[1] UK Department of Health, Start Active Stay Active (July 2011), p10

Being obese can increase the risk of developing a range of serious diseases, including hypertension, type 2 diabetes, cardiovascular diseases, several cancers, asthma, obstructive sleep apnea, and musculoskeletal problem.[2] There are plenty of diets to choose from, but only certain ones will help you get other health problems under control. Diets that target specific health conditions or diseases can make it easier on your body to lose the weight because the diet is focused on whole body health.

By selecting a diet that treats the whole body, you're more likely to have long term success because you'll be getting and feeling healthier as you lose weight. The focus of a diet that shows you how to eat well and get fit will be on improving your lifestyle rather than as a quick fix.

Allergies and Gut Issues

A conflict I have found with many diet plans is an ignorance of allergies or the variety of gut issues from Celiac Disease to IBS. When a diet is restricted to very specific foods or to meal supplements, finding alternatives to a food allergy or sensitivity you may have becomes almost impossible.

You need to pay close attention to your diet plan making sure that you get the balances of

---

[2] Public Health England (IDH0063) para 15

nutrients and food types while also including only those foods that agree with your individual system.

There is a lot of advice and opinion out there about the wide variety of gut issues which cause people to suffer. Most of information you are going to find has no scientific base or at best very suspect scientific data. The best thing you can do is to listen to your own body, and your trusted health professional. The one sure thing is that staying away from processed food will help. Oddly, some foods can help reduce allergic or sensitivity reactions. There's some truth to the saying that an apple a day keeps the doctor away. Apples are good in diets for allergies and so are red grapes. Nuts, onions and garlic can also fight allergies. Turmeric, especially as a supplement, can help reduce inflammation, swelling, and other allergic reactions. Look for a diet that includes these helpful foods, assuming, of course, you aren't allergic to those foods.

Heart Disease

A lot of people struggle with health issues that can cause heart disease. One of the symptoms of this health issue early on can be high blood pressure readings. If you have a problem keeping your blood pressure under good control, you'll want to look for a diet that can help you with that.

One of those diets is the DASH diet. This is an acronym for Dietary Approach to Stop Hypertension and it's one of the diets that the National Institutes of Health recommends for people who have hypertension.

You can either use the regular DASH eating plan or the one that's geared toward lowered sodium meals. There are no special foods to buy. You simply eat healthy ones, like fruits and vegetables, low fat dairy and lean meats.

You can learn more about the DASH diet from the Mayo Clinic online.

If the DASH plan isn't what you wanted, there are other diet plans beneficial to heart disease reversal and prevention. Other diets beneficial for the heart are the TLC diet, Flexitarian diets, a vegan or vegetarian diet, and many more.

The Mayo Clinic and WebMD online are information dense on several of these diets to help you decide which might fit your lifestyle choices and healthy requirements.

Diabetes

Another health issue you want to look at when you're searching for the right diet plan for you is your glucose control. If you've been diagnosed with pre-diabetes or diabetes, you want that stabilized to either prevent getting full blown diabetes or getting it under control to stave off long term health affects that diabetes can sometimes cause.

Exercise seems to be of particular importance when combating diabetes. By choosing a diet plan that promotes exercising, you can bring your diabetes under control and have A1c levels within recommended ranges.

You can use the DASH diet for treating diabetes as well, but any other healthy diet specific for treating this condition is fine.

If you don't want to try the DASH diet, there are others, including the Engine 2 diet, the Mayo Clinic diet, the Glycemic Index diet and more. What each of these plans have in common is a focus on lifestyle changes for the long term. They all have similar takeaways, they all encourage more plant-based, fresh food options and they all seek to increase the activity levels in your day to day routine.

Some lessons you can learn from each of these and similar diet/healthy lifestyle plans are:

- Be mindful while you are eating; don't watch TV during a meal
- Set realistic goals you can commit to in this moment
- Eat unprocessed fresh food as much as possible
- Eat out less, eat at home more
- Be active, move

Anti-Aging

The foods that you eat can take a toll on your organs. If you eat a diet that's high in fat and red meats, not only does it show up on your skin, but it can cause cellular aging within the body, too.

Diets that can help with anti-aging have one thing in common. The diet is centered on foods that are natural and will result in a safe rate of weight loss. The foods in any anti-aging diet will include whole grains because fiber helps your blood vessels stay in good shape.

A diet that's rich with anti-aging properties will also have fish and lean meats as the protein suggestions for your meals. Fish is rich in Omega-3 and can also assist users with maintaining cognitive skills including fighting against memory loss.

The anti-aging diet will also have you eating plenty of antioxidant bearing fruits and vegetables. Not only do you get the benefit of eating foods that help in the fight against cancer, but these foods help your eyes fight against conditions that would attack your eyesight.

If aging too rapidly is a concern for you, here are some additional lifestyle steps to consider:

- Get enough restful sleep
- Stretch; I use, and recommend, Somatic Exercise

- Move
- Reduce sugars, including those found in alcohol
- Yoga, for balance and strength
- Weight bearing exercise, for bone strength
- Acceptance and celebration of aging with grace

Inflammation

Some people struggle with inflammation, and it is a big part of what affects the aging process as well. Whether it's short or long term, inflammation in the body can make you feel miserable. You want to have an eating plan that will give your body relief from inflammation. Diets that contain sugary foods or foods that are high in saturated fats can trigger certain inflammation. If you've been struggling with any kind of inflammatory disease or you have arthritis in your joints that seems to get worse, what you're eating could be what's triggering your flare ups.

Diets that help treat inflammations are diets that suggest avoiding white foods like sugar and white flour. Vegetarian and flexitarian diets are good diets for people who have inflammation. Even eating a vegetarian meal plan a few times a week can make a difference in how you feel. Any foods that are good as part of a balanced meal will help you lose weight, but you'll notice that you feel better when you eat foods that target inflammation.

One of the diets that you might want to check out if you're struggling with inflammation or arthritis is the Paleo diet. Fair warning though with Paleo, there are a lot of variations out there, the premise of the diet being genetically based is BS, and it is not designed for weight loss. That said if you can control portions and be thoughtful about what you consume you will feel better on a Paleo style diet.

Lots of the foods that are anti-aging are also anti-inflammatory, here are some examples:

- Blueberries
- Almonds
- Oats
- Dark chocolate
- Green tea
- Ginger
- Turmeric
- Wild salmon
- Broccoli
- Beets
- Red peppers
- Back Beans
- Tomatoes
- Spinach
- Pineapple
- Eggs
- Whole grains

- Yogurt
- Apples
- Garlic
- Oysters
- Tuna
- Rosemary
- Bone broth

Cancer Prevention

The right diet can help prevent cancer. Did you know that after smoking, obesity may be the second greatest preventable cause of cancer? "Research has shown that many types of cancer are more common in people who are overweight or obese, including cancers of the breast (in women after menopause), bowel, womb, oesophageal (food pipe), pancreatic, kidney, liver, upper stomach (gastric cardia), gallbladder, ovarian, thyroid, myeloma (a type of blood cancer), and meningioma (a type of brain tumour)."[3]

The increased risk is because of the hormones and proteins released by fat cells and traveling throughout the body. Fat cells can attract immune cells to body tissues. These immune cells release chemicals that cause long-lasting inflammation which can raise the risk of cancer.

---

[3] cancerresearchuk.org/about-cancer/causes-of-cancer/bodyweight-and-cancer/how-being-overweight-causes-cancer

There are foods that can boost your ability to fight cancer too!

Look for diets that will help your body give you a boost up on cancer prevention. The American Journal of Clinical Nutrition published a story that showed the benefits of the Mediterranean diet against the risk of getting breast cancer. In this diet, users avoid the saturated fats and processed foods that contain ingredients that aren't good for the body. Instead, people who follow the Mediterranean diet can help keep cancer at bay by eating foods rich in antioxidants and fish containing Omega 3.

If you're looking for a diet that will give you long term benefits, this is a good one, especially if you have a family history of certain cancers.

Energy

If you seem to struggle with not having enough energy to get through the day, you'll want to look for a diet that can help to boost your energy levels. The kinds of diets that can help you to get your stamina back are diets that are loaded with high fiber foods and foods that help keep your energy level up during your waking hours.

If you're looking to boost your energy, then you need to be careful around low carb diets because carbs give you energy and the more complex the carb, the higher amount of energy it gives you as it turns the carb into fuel for your body.

If energy is a side health issue for you, then you might benefit from a diet plan that requires multiple small meals throughout the day. That helps keep your metabolism boosted so that you can function better.

Energy comes from complex carbohydrates, proteins, and fats. Make sure you are getting complex carbohydrates, and healthy fats. If you are using any of the diet plans already mentioned, you are very likely getting the proper mix of these three energy manufacturers. *Still suffering from low cyclical energy?*

There may be a very easy fix. Water!

What if you are already staying completely away from sodas and sweets, limiting your alcohol and caffeine consumption? The question to ask is are you getting enough fluids? Drink water, and then drink some more water.

Dehydration lowers energy, makes the body inefficient, and can even affect mood and cognitive function.

Drink water all day long!

Infertility and Menstrual Cycles

Carrying too much extra weight can make it more difficult to conceive. If you need to lose weight and you're struggling with infertility, there are diets that can help you with that health issue.

Certain foods affect your hormonal levels and can help you with ovulation. The nutrients in some foods play a role in your reproductive ability and your hormones need these nutrients for you to conceive. According to a Harvard Study, a high "fertility diet" score was characterized by a lower intake of trans fat with a simultaneous greater intake of monounsaturated fat; a lower intake of animal protein with greater vegetable protein intake; a higher intake of high-fiber, low-glycemic carbohydrates; greater preference for high-fat dairy products; higher nonheme iron intake; and higher frequency of multivitamin use.[4]

You will want a diet that's rich in green, red and yellow vegetables and you want to choose organic foods whenever possible. Eat a lot of fish and stay away from processed foods.

Get your servings of fiber because that helps your hormones get the balance that they need. A good example of a diet for infertility would again be the Mediterranean diet.

Other Health Concerns

Sometimes habits we have can really do a number on our health. But there are diets that can help us stop continuing with bad habits. Smoking can be curbed through a sound diet

[4] Diet and Lifestyle in the Prevention of Ovulatory Disorder Infertility
Chavarro, Jorge E. MD, ScD1,2; Rich-Edwards, Janet W. MPH, ScD2,3,4; Rosner, Bernard A. PhD2,5; Willett, Walter C. MD, DrPH1,2,4
Obstetrics & Gynecology: November 2007 - Volume 110 - Issue 5 - pp 1050-1058
doi: 10.1097/01.AOG.00 0287293.25465.e1

and the foods in a healthy diet can help repair damage done to the body from smoking.

To stop smoking, look for a diet that offers plenty of hard, crunchy food. Some foods that aren't good for you will make smoking taste better, while other foods, such as apples, make a cigarette taste worse.

Stress is another health issue with which many people deal. There are diets that can help you fight stress. These diets suggest stress fighting foods such as oatmeal, complex carbs, fruits and vegetables.

Indigestion is never fun. Normally, a diet that suggests lots of fruits and vegetables is beneficial for all users, but not for people with indigestion. If you suffer from this, you'll want to stay away from diets that are filled with acidic foods, which worsen indigestion.

Avoid citric and tomato-based foods as well as coffee, garlic and spicy foods. Sometimes, you'll only need to cut them out in the evening hours, but you can enjoy them early in the day.

If you want to leave insomnia behind, you can do it naturally through diet. There are foods that contain tryptophan, which helps you sleep. Diets high in whole grain foods, fruits and vegetables and low-fat dairy products can help you stop tossing and turning.

If you want a diet that helps you heal from skin problems, diets that are heavy in fish, especially salmon, can help. Blueberries are great at correcting skin problems, too.

You want to avoid pineapples because they can cause flare-ups and so can certain spices. Diets that focus on spices as a way of preparing meals wouldn't be good for you.

Did you know that certain foods can trigger a headache? They can! Some foods contain tyramine and can bring on a headache. Foods containing tyramine are processed meats, beans, soups, nuts and many cheeses. If you suffer from headaches, do a little elimination test with these foods and see if you can pinpoint the culprit.

You never want to choose a diet plan solely based on how many pounds it can help you whittle off your body in the shortest amount of time. Instead, you want to look good and feel great!

You want longevity and good health with your new, trim figure. It's important that you base your diet plan choices on its health-benefiting traits according to what you need for your body!

Now What?

It is time to set some goals for your healthy lifestyle. Pick and choose a diet framework that works for your goals and health needs. Embrace a plan for movement, activity and exercise that sounds like fun and fits your schedule and personality.

What are your top three goals for a healthier you?

What are the obstacles that could keep you from achieving these goals?

How will you overcome those obstacles?

I am here to help if you need me. I have a service plan focused on helping you become your healthiest self. I am happy to offer you recipes and suggestions to further your journey and success. In fact, as a bonus, below is recipe for bone broth that is amazingly tasty!

Contact me at challberg@dogwatchnavigation.com or visit the website to learn more. Please let me know how you are doing on your journey; I'd love to hear about your victories big and small.

Bone Broth

4 quarts of water

1 teaspoon salt

2 tablespoons apple cider vinegar

2 large onions, unpeeled and coarsely chopped

2 carrots, scrubbed and coarsely chopped

3 celery stalks with leaves, coarsely chopped

1 bunch fresh flat leave parsley

3 or 4 garlic cloves, lightly smashed

4 # meat beef bones

1 lemon, sliced lengthwise

6 whole peppercorns

Shake of sea salt

Place the bones on a cookie sheet and roast at a low temperature for 30 minutes. Place the bones in a large slow cooker with the water and the vinegar. Let it just soak for a few minutes. Place the rest of the ingredients in the slow cooker (you might want to bundle the parsley) and turn onto high until it comes to a boil. Reduce the setting to low and cook for 12 to 24 hours. The longer it cooks, the better it tastes! Stain the stock through a fine mesh strainer or a coffee filter, after removing the parsley bundle, into a large bowl. Discard the waste.

Be healthy!

Go ahead! Write some notes…

www.ingramcontent.com/pod-product-compliance
Lightning Source LLC
Chambersburg PA
CBHW020331290526
45785CB00007B/3007